PERSONAL JOURNAL
&
RECIPES FOR HEALTHY LIVING

2020 Edition

Renee Alter

Disclaimer

The information, including but not limited to, text, graphics, images, and other material contained in this book are for informational purposes only. The purpose of this book is to promote broad consumer under-standing and knowledge of various health related topics. It is not intended to be a substitute for professional medical advice, diagnosis, or treatment. Always seek the advice of your physician or other qualified health care provider with any questions you may have regarding any medical condition or treatment and before undertaking a new health care regimen, and never disregard professional medical advice or delay in seeking it because of something you have read in this book.

The techniques and advice described in this book represent the opinions of the author based on her training and experience. The author expressly dis-claims any responsibility for any liability, loss, or risk, personal or otherwise, which is incurred as a result of using any of the techniques, recipes, or recommendations suggested herein. If in any doubt, or if requiring medical advice, please contact the appropriate health professional.

The author has made every effort to provide accurate internet addresses at the time of publication. Further-more, the author does not have any control over and does not assume any responsibility for author or third-party websites or their content.

SELF REFLECTION

IS THE KEY

TO

PERSONAL GROWTH

Table of Contents

Introduction

The purpose of this journal is to assist you with all aspects of your life, beginning with revisiting your childhood and reconnecting to the playful, adventurous part of yourself who dreamed big dreams and had an amazing imagination. I, as the author, encourage you to go on the journey. This isn't about feeling bad about what happened if bad things did happen. This is about exploring what conclusions you made as a result of your life circumstances and learning to acknowledge, love, accept, forgive, and move the stagnant subconscious energies out of your mind and out of your body.

We all are traveling an amazing journey of self-discovery. There are always new life lessons to learn. Shifting your beliefs about all things earthly can transform your life. We become who we think we will become. We develop beliefs that do not serve us, our higher good, or the good of our planet.

There are many self-help books out there. I know. I've read a LOT of them. I even included some of the titles in this book. I wanted something simple with few words but big impact. I wanted a book that could be a companion guide for upcoming workshops when I succeed in putting them together.

For those who are thinking about writing a memoir, this book can help you organize your thoughts and provide a foundation for you to begin.

Rise and Shine!

Today is the first day of the rest of your life!

Yesterday is gone… let it go. It can only live in your memories. Keep the good ones and release ones that don't serve you.

Take a deep breath. Inhale in one second intervals for six (6), hold for 20-30 seconds, exhale with a shhhh like you are telling someone to be quiet. Do this until you feel a nice buzz. You can also exhale with a haaaaa and feel the air move up through your throat.

Next, brush your teeth… but not with over-the-counter fluoride toothpaste with toxic chemicals.

Now drink an eight (8) ounce glass of water. If you can tolerate it, a spoonful of Organic ACV (Apple Cider Vinegar) is an added health benefit.

Download Plant Nanny from Google Play Store. Watch adorable plants grow while you are being reminded to drink water. The app calculates how much water you need per your weight and other stats.

You are ready to start your day!

Set an intention such as: I intend to have a wonderful day!

Serenity Prayer

God grant me the serenity…

Serenity means that I no longer recoil from the past, live in jeopardy because of my present behavior, or worry about the unknown future. I seek regular times to re-create myself and I avoid those times of depletion that make me vulnerable to despair and to old self-destructive patterns.

…to accept the things I cannot change…

Accepting change means that I do not cause suffering for myself by clinging to that which no longer exists. All that I can count on is that nothing will be stable—except how I respond to the transforming cycles in my life of birth, growth, and death.

…the courage to change the things I can…

Giving up my attempts to control outcomes does not require that I give up my boundaries or my best efforts. It does mean my most honest appraisal of the limits of what I can do.

…and the wisdom to know the difference.
Wisdom becomes the never forgotten recognition of all those times when it seemed there was no way out, and new paths opened up like miracles in my life.

Note: Received from a recovering alcoholic who got this from AA.

Essential Elements
for a Life Lived Well

O xygen – Breathe Deeply (7 x's)

W ater – Drink ½ your weight in ounces

N utrition – Protein, Fruits, Vegetables

E nergy - Exercise

R elaxation / **Restoration** – BEing vs. DOing

S exual Intimacy – Close friends & family (hugs)

H eat – Sunlight / direct sun

I ntestinal Elimination – Stay regular

P leasure & Pain – Power of 3 (Gratitude)

Note: Based on OWNERSHIP and the SOULDIERS S6 Sequence by Jaramy Eugene Wilson.

Rituals for Thriving

- Exercise
- Meditate / Breathe
- Journal / Write
- Dance
- Go on a date (even if you're married)
- Connect with nature
- Visualize
- Family Time
- Cook / Eat a healthy meal
- Organize your space / life
- Get rid of things I don't love
- Be with friends
- Play
- Let go / Forgive
- Sing / Make music
- Create Art
- Read for enjoyment
- Connect / Pray
- Call someone / Write a letter
- Stretch / Do Yoga
- Massage / Exchange touch
- Serve my community

Note: I got this from thedragontree.com, however their journal was way too complex for what I needed. Just in case it is what YOU would like to have, visit this website to purchase it.

YOU ARE
A SHINING STAR!

Setting Goals

Failing to plan is planning to fail. If you don't set goals or make a plan, life will happen to you instead of you intentionally creating the life you want.

There are many types of goal-setting techniques. One is S.M.A.R.T. Specific, Measurable, Achievable, Realistic, and Time-Bound. This is the general business plan but can work in other aspects of your life as well.

Another method is dividing your goals up according to your values. Determine what you value. Categories can include: Spiritual, Family, Emotional, Financial, Career, Physical (Health), Social, Relationships, Education.

Stephen Covey divides up goals by roles. He suggests you 1) Connect to a Mission 2) Review Roles 3) Identify Goals 4) Organize Weekly. What roles do you play in life? Parent, Co-Worker, Business Owner, Author, Volunteer, Husband, Wife, Sister, Brother, you get the idea.

Create a Vision / Mission Statement for how you want to live your life. Most businesses and non-profits have one. This will help you get clear on what you value most so you can decide which things / tasks to pursue and which to let go of.

Type *Goal Setting* in Amazon and there are hundreds of books on the topic. One of my favorites is:

7 Habits of Highly Effective People by Stephen Covey

Decisions, Decisions, Decisions

Feeling overwhelmed? Don't know what to do?

Ask yourself, "What is really important right now?" Think of the situation as either a wooden ball or a crystal ball. There are just some things you can't afford to drop.

Think about the long-term outcome you want to have. Which task/option will get you there? Put the rest on your Someday List. There's more than one way to 'skin a cat,' but you don't have to do everything at once... or do it perfectly.

Go through each option. First imagine having or experiencing that thing. Then imagine not having or experiencing that thing. In both cases, notice your gut reaction.

Sleep on it. If you do all the things above and just can't figure something out, before you go to sleep, say a prayer asking for divine guidance and set an intention for your subconscious to get the answer while you sleep. Keep a notepad and pen by your bed so you can capture the answers as you wake up, even if it is in the middle of the night.

Note: This general message was originally written by Jewell Siebert. I've reworded it to fit on one page. I've personally met Jewell, and she is an amazing Life Coach, trained under Jack Canfield. For more about Jewell, go to: http://jewellsiebert.com

Goals For This Year

Long-Term Life Goals

Milestones & Achievements

Books I Read

Note: Authors appreciate reviews on their books. Please leave reviews on Amazon or any other site they are published through (like Smashwords).

Movies I Watched / Went To See

15

SAVE THE BEES. WITHOUT THEM, OUR FOOD SUPPLY IS IN DANGER.

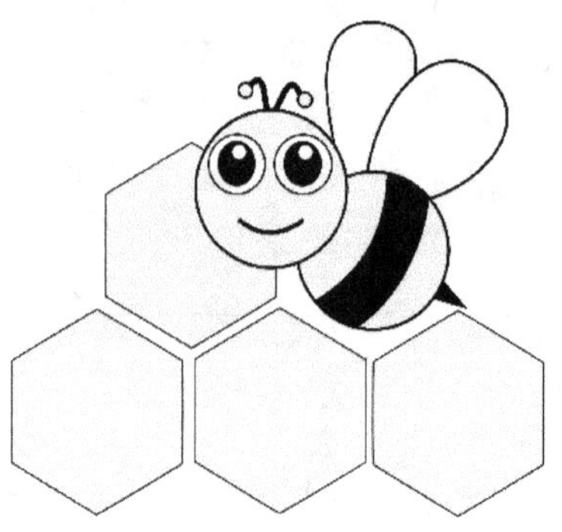

16

Mental Health

Are you feeling blah? Before you get a prescription for antidepressants, consider the following.

STRESS will mess you up! Our modern world is filled with it. The caveman tigers that only set off the fight or flight response occasionally are now present 24/7 if you let them. Your body can't reset, heal, and recharge while you are in this state.

Your thoughts can mess you up, too. (See next page).

There are new studies that show serotonin is produced in your gut. As you up the level of nutrition, eliminate toxins and the Standard American Diet aka SAD (ironically when you eat these foods you DO become SAD), get restorative sleep, stay socially connected, reduce stress, your moods will improve. See a complimentary or alternative medicine practitioner to identify nutritional deficiencies.

Vianna Stibal wrote *Theta Healing* and *Advanced Theta Healing* after discovering people weren't getting well because of subconscious beliefs. These books list just about every emotion / belief on the planet. When you read them and see yourself in there, you will no longer feel so alone.

If you are feeling the isolation of depression, author John Clark III wrote *Depression Blues* and has a website where you can get this book as a free download.

http://depressionblues.net/

Watch Your Thoughts

Most people are unaware of the thousands of thoughts that compete for space in their minds all day of every day, continuing while they sleep. And most of these thoughts find hiding places in your subconscious where they seem to make up rules about how to implement them in your life. Thoughts are powerful. Learning to manage them is a must.

Awareness is the ability to directly know and perceive, to feel, or to be cognizant of events. More broadly, it is the state or quality of being conscious of something. (Wikipedia).

On the next page is a list of 10 Cognitive Distortions otherwise known as the 10 Forms of Twisted Thinking. Most people have at least some of them.

<u>Books to read</u>:

I AM by Stephen Shaw

Feeling Good: The New Mood Therapy by David Burns, M.D.

The Biology of Belief by Bruce Lipton, Ph.D.

Managing Your Mind by Gillian Butler, Ph.D. & Tony Hope, M.D.

The Miracle Morning by Hal Elrod

Hal Elrod on YouTube:
https://www.youtube.com/watch?v=U0uRp7BoPVY

10 Cognitive Distortions

All or nothing thinking: (seeing things as either black or white, good or bad)

Overgeneralization: (seeing a single negative event as a never-ending pattern of defeat)

Mental filter: (picking out a single negative detail and dwelling on it exclusively so that your vision of all of reality becomes darkened)

Discounting the positive: (rejecting positive experiences by insisting they don't count)

Jumping to conclusions: (you interpret things negatively when there are no facts to support your conclusion)

Magnification: (exaggerating the importance of your problems and shortcomings)

Emotional reasoning: (assuming your negative emotions reflect the way things really are)

Should statements: (telling yourself that things SHOULD be the way you hoped or expected them to be)

Labeling: (the extreme of all or nothing thinking)

Personalization and blame: (holding yourself responsible for events that aren't entirely under your control or doing the opposite and blaming other people or circumstances for your problems)

Note: From *Feeling Good: The New Mood Therapy*

Thoughts I Can Work On Reframing

Take note of your thoughts throughout the day. How do they fit into one of the categories in the 10 Cognitive Distortions? Here is where you'll begin to untwist your thinking and learn how reframe.

How I Want To Feel

What I want to feel less of vs. what I want to feel more of

Disinterested, Bored, Distressed, Somber, Discouraged, Gloomy	Optimistic, Cheerful, Happy, Lighthearted, Resilient, Enthusiastic *(Cheer-Uplifting Blend)*
Apathetic, Discouraged, Gloomy, Anxious, Insecure, Distressed	Confidence, Courage, Belief, Trust, Energy, Drive *(Motivate-Encouraging Blend)*
Somber, Disinterested, Bored, Discontented, Bitter, Angry	Daring, Passionate, Joyful, Excited, Spontaneous, Creative, Inspired *(Passion-Inspiring Blend)*
Discontented, Bitter, Angry, Ashamed, Sad, Grieving	Contented, Relieved, Charitable, Patient, Accepting, Gracious *(Forgive-Renewing Blend)*
Ashamed, Sad, Grieving, Hurt, Worried, Fearful	Hopeful, Sustained, Whole, Comforted, Reconciled, Revived *(Console-Comforting Blend)*
Hurt, Worried, Fearful, Anxious, Insecure, Apathetic	Composed, Centered, At Ease, Brave, Calm, Reassured *(Peace-Reassuring Blend)*

Note: From doTERRA's Emotional Aroma Therapy Kit

<u>Cells</u>

Once upon a time, you were a single cell. Everything you needed for life existed in this cell. This single cell had innate intelligence and knew what to do to become a human being with over 50 trillion cells, incredibly laid out into an amazing universe of organs, bone, nerves, brain, arteries, veins, etc.

In Bruce Lipton's book, *The Biology of Belief*, he wrote about this miracle and all his discoveries, including the fact that cells are affected by their environment. Environment includes thoughts, beliefs, and emotions. He discovered genes do NOT control our destiny – the environment does.

Knowing this, isn't the human body truly even more miraculous than you ever thought it could be? There is a video on YouTube *Admire the perfect creation of God*. Watch it. You are a miracle. It's time you treated yourself like one.

There's a lot of new info about the mitochondria of cells. Mitochondria are your cellular batteries. When you start from the very beginning, your health depends on the health of Mito. Caution: drugs damage Mito. *They are organelles that act like a digestive system which takes in nutrients, breaks them down, and creates energy rich molecules for the cell. Many of the reactions involved in cellular respiration happen in the mitochondria. Mitochondria are the working organelles that keep the cell full of energy.* (Biology4Kids.com)

Parenting

Now that you were introduced to a cell and how it became you, where are you at regarding parenting? Are you already a parent? Married? Divorced? Single Parent? Wouldn't it have been nice if we had parenting classes in high school? Do you think you had great parents? Abusive parents? Alcoholic or drug addict parents? Given up for adoption? Did one or both parents die when you were young?

Contemplate how parenting has affected you, how parenting affected your parents, and who you are as a parent if you are one. What were the strengths? What were the weaknesses? What is most memorable (both good and bad)? Write your thoughts on these questions below.

<u>Age 2</u>

Try to imagine your life when you were two years old. The goal here is to figure out what beliefs you developed before you were old enough to realize what you decided to believe wasn't necessarily true. What were your parents' life like while your mother was pregnant? Were your parents in love? Were they unhappy? Were they together? Apart? Are you aware you would have been affected by your mother's stress, illness, or mental illness such as depression?

Notes to My 2-Year-Old Self

Basic Nutrition

YOU ARE WHAT YOU EAT!

<u>Protein</u>: Grass Fed Meat, Pasture-Raised Poultry/Eggs, Alaskan Wild Caught Omega 3 Fish, Raw Nuts, Seeds.

<u>Fruits & Vegetables</u>: Go to Environmental Working Group's website at ewg.org for the current list of the Clean 15 and the Dirty Dozen.

<u>Beans & Lentils</u>: If you are not on a Paleo plan, Harmony House has great fully cooked dehydrated organic that will be ready to eat in about 10-15 minutes after adding hot water. Even better is cooking beans in a pressure cooker (Instant Pot) to reduce lectins.

<u>Fats</u>: Avocado, Avocado Oil, Coconut Oil, Olive Oil, Grass Fed Butter, Sesame Oil, Walnut Oil, Flax Seed Oil. Avoid saturated fats, trans fats, and Omega 6 oils such as corn, safflower, sunflower, canola, palm, soybean, and peanut oils.

<u>Minerals</u>: Himalayan Pink Salt or Rock Salt or Balanced Ionic Minerals.

<u>Water</u>: Drink half of your weight in ounces. Mountain Spring Water is best.

<u>Chocolate</u>: Buy unprocessed high percent (85%) cacao which is high in bioflavonoids. Place a square on the roof of your mouth and let it dissolve. The nutrients will go directly into your brain! My favorite brand is *Green & Black's*.

FOOD IS EITHER YOUR SUSTENANCE OR YOUR POISON

<u>Consider the following</u>:

<u>Salt</u>: Before the age of refrigeration, meat was preserved in salt – the original. We got all the minerals we needed. The minerals were then processed out of the salt to keep it from clumping. When people got Goiters, iodine was added back in, but without all the other minerals, it threw us out of balance. Our cells communicate *electrically*.

<u>Wheat</u>: Wheat grown today is not the same as what was grown a hundred years ago or more. Not only has it been genetically modified, but before it is collected from the fields with tractors, it is doused with Roundup to kill it all, so it won't glue up the tractors. In addition to the Roundup, flour used for baking is processed and *bromine* (a neurotoxin) is added to keep it from clumping. Bromine is also sprayed on berries to keep them from getting moldy.

<u>Gluten</u>: Many people are gluten sensitive and don't even know it. Gluten is not just in food. It is also in makeup, lotions, and other skincare products.

<u>Lectins</u>: According to Dr. Peter Osborne (*No Grain, No Pain*), any food that has lectins will be difficult to digest for people who have compromised guts and auto-immune issues. (Gluten is just one type of lectin.)

Gluten-Free: Read the ingredients of prepackaged gluten-free products. They often include many of the ingredients that should be avoided. Better to make your own.

Corn & Soy: Most of it is genetically modified to grow despite being doused with Roundup. Fermented soy is best.

Cows and Pigs: Unless they are personally farm raised, animals are injected with hormones so they will grow FAST. So fast, that I heard a local farmer say their pig had to be 'processed' before it got any bigger. They are also given antibiotics to deter disease in crowded conditions. Watch *Food, Inc. Full Movie* on YouTube. You'll get the idea. These animals are fed the above GMO corn and soy. Milk from these cows have said hormones and antibiotics in it, too. If you ARE raising your own, beware of feeding them grains, especially the GMO corn and soy.

Yogurt: Yogurts with fruit, berries, etc. are very high in sugar. It also most likely comes from cows in the section mentioned above... fed grains and injected with anti-biotics and hormones. If you can tolerate dairy, it is best to make your own.

Sugar: It has been added to most processed foods, including above yogurt. This sugar has also been processed. Fortunately, you can buy Black Strap Molasses, the part that has the minerals and nutrients processed out of the original form of sugar. Organic is rich in calcium and magnesium.

Chocolate: The original form of chocolate has many health benefits. Chocolate that is processed (with alkali) no longer has any nutritional value. It is also most likely contaminated with lead. (Dr. Mercola)

Soda: Diet sodas meant to be calorie free can CAUSE weight gain. See Artificial Sweeteners.

Artificial Sweeteners: Every chemical your body doesn't recognize *is stored in fat cells*. Your body doesn't recognize ANY of the artificial sweeteners. Sadly, it is in a LOT of packaged food, especially the 'sugar-free' ones.

Fats: Ever since the FDA promoted margarine, canola oil, and other unhealthy vegetable oils high in Omega 6 fats, obesity and related health issues have soared. Healthy fats are higher in Omega 3 than Omega 6. Some of them are Olive Oil, Avocado Oil, and Coconut Oil. Cows raised on grains instead of grass are high in Omega 6 fats. The only oil that does not go rancid when heated is Coconut oil.

Recommended Reading – See Reading List for Health

Healthy Snacks

Fresh Fruit + Raw Nuts

Dried Fruit + Raw Nuts

Frozen organic melon balls (Watermelon or Honeydew/Cantaloupe combo)

Crunchy vegetables like Jicama & Carrots dipped in a Wholly Guacamole single serving packet.

Cook sweet potatoes ahead of time and eat with pecans (pretend it is Pecan Pie)

Quick pick-me-up – Dark Chocolate (melt a square on the roof of your mouth & it will go directly into your brain)

Also snack on the following:

Singing
Reading
Walking
Hugging
Sprinting
Socializing
Family Time
Listen to Music
Knitting / Sewing
Playing an Instrument

Sense of Smell

Humans are very much affected by their sense of smell. You determine what you will eat by what it smells like. You know you need a bath when you smell stinky. You know your DOG needs a bath when it smells stinky. You may have cedar fever or are allergic to mold. Your refrigerator may have spoiled food. Your house may smell musty.

"Also known as CN1, the olfactory nerve is the first of 12 cranial nerves located within the head. It relays sensory data to the brain, and it is responsible for the sense of smell." (Health Line)

There are many smells that are toxic, such as ingredients in cleaners and certain types of mold.

Many essential oils have been proven to influence your moods. There are individual oils and oil blends for every possible mood. Consider getting an ultrasonic diffuser and filling your home, office, or classroom (if you're a teacher) with heavenly scents. Caution: some essential oils are poisonous to pets. And take time to go outside and…

AND SMELL THE ROSES!

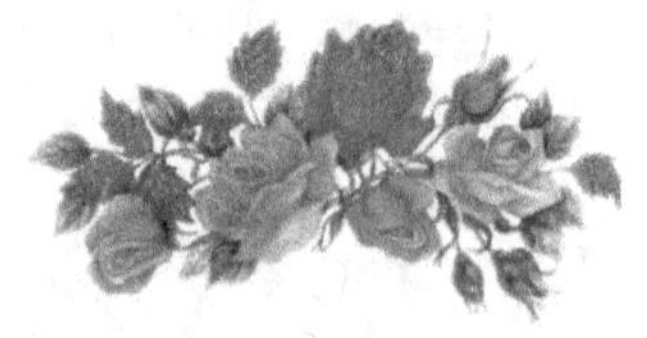

<u>Grounding</u>

When you were a child, I bet you laid out in the grass and felt the earth move beneath you. You were grounding to the energies of the earth. Earth is alive and breathing and in this complex high-tech life, we are suffering from too much EMF's from electronic gadgets. When was the last time you even stood barefoot in the grass or on the beach? If you don't like to be barefoot (fire ants in Texas), there are grounding shoes and mats. River rocks can ground you, too.

"Our bodies and cells have electrical energy, and especially with the high prevalence of Electromagnetic waves, Wi-Fi and mobile phone waves, many of us have a high amount of positive electrons built up in our bodies." (Wellness Mama)

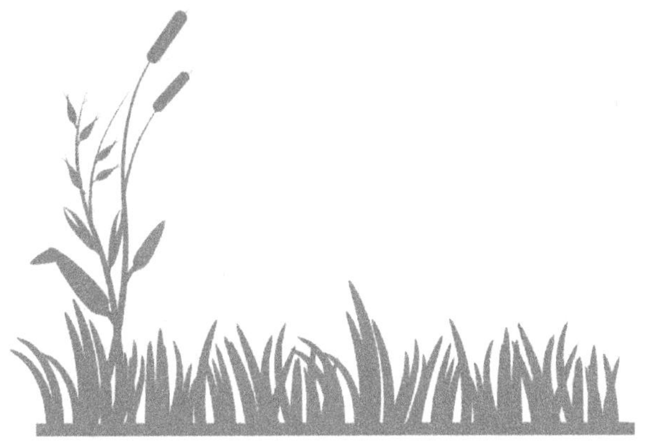

<u>Book to read</u>: *Earthing: The Most Important Health Discovery Ever* by Clinton Ober and Dr. Stephen T Sinatra M.D.

<u>Photo Page</u>

Find a photo of you when you were about five years old and place it here. Wasn't this child cute? Adorable? Smart? Creative? Playful? Loveable? This child will always live inside of you. I bet when you look at him/her, he/she could do no wrong. You knew this child could not intentionally do anything evil or bad. If you have or had a child of your own, I'm pretty sure you viewed them very differently than how you view your-self – the part of you that is still this child. Visualize a time in your life when felt really happy. What were you doing?

<u>Age 6</u>

By the time you are six years old, your identity has been formed. You believe whatever you were taught to believe. Question everything. Many have decided they will never be good enough, smart enough, or worthy of love, which will affect them for the rest of their lives – until they realize what happened and make the decision to work on themselves and grow past this. Refer to the list of Cognitive Distortions. Who did you decide you were when you were six years old?

Notes to My 6-Year-Old Self

Things I Liked to Do When I Was 6

<u>Teenager</u>

The year you turn 13 marks a major milestone. You are now a teenager. There are many cultural traditions performed as a rite of passage, some at age 13, others before and after. Here are two of them:

- Jewish Coming of Age Tradition age 12-13: Bar and Bat Mitzvah
- In the Brazilian Amazon, young boys belonging to the indigenous Sateré-Mawé tribe mark their coming of age when they turn 13 in a Bullet and Ant Initiation

YOU ARE LOVED
JUST THE WAY YOU ARE!

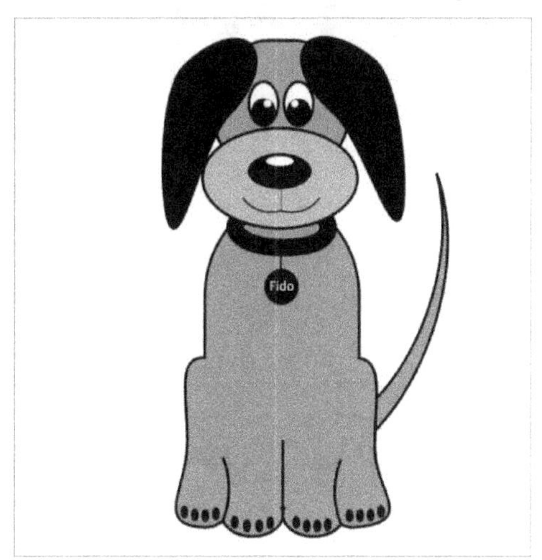

Things I Liked to Do When I Was 13

Friends can be your pets, too. If you didn't have any friends or only had one, don't feel sad…

THINK WARM FUZZY THOUGHTS

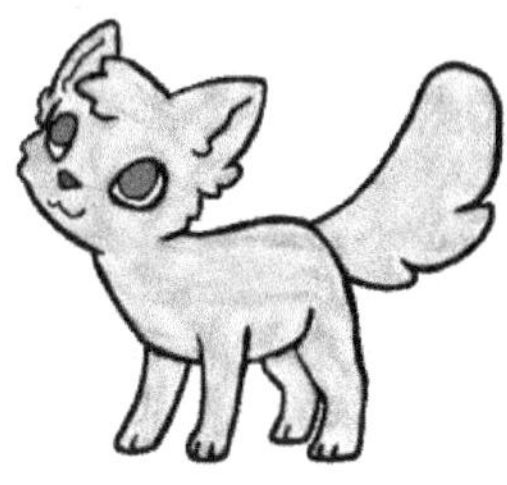

Notes to My 13-Year-Old Self

If I Were 13 Again, I'd…

My Favorite Subjects & Career Ideas

Some people know at a young age what they want to be when they grow up. Some are more creative and adventurous and want to try many things. Boys may not figure out what they want to do until they are 25. Some people work for family business. Some join the military. Some do what their families expect them to do, but their unhappiness takes a toll on their health. Are you doing what you wanted to do at 13? Did you know what you wanted to do when you were 13?

Egg Loaf

Mix ¾ cup Harmony House Vegetable Soup Mix and
2 TBSP ground flax seeds in ¾ cup of water.
Put aside to hydrate.

Combine ¾ cup almond flour and
¼ cup mesquite bean flour.

Scramble 4 eggs.

When veggie mix and flax seeds have absorbed the
water, mix all the ingredients together. Add a little
more water if needed.

Use batter to make pancakes or muffins or
a loaf. I like using 3 small Pyrex loaf pans in my
toaster oven at 375° for 30 minutes. Cool. Use a small
rubber spatula between loaf and pan on all sides and
slide rubber spatula under the loaves to release them
from the bottom. Freeze leftovers.

Note: Harmony House grows organic vegetables and
dehydrates them, which are sold on Amazon in quart
and gallon containers. Choose eggs from pasture-raised
chickens (that were not fed grains). In the documentary
Food, Inc., chickens are shown to be crowded into dark
metal barns and fed GMO corn and soy. Chickens raised
to roam free eat bugs and healthier feed, so they are
higher in Omega 3's.

<u>Relationships</u>

Infatuation and unconditional love are very different things. With infatuation, you think you're in love, but what you are really in love with is the IDEA of what the other person (or thing) can bring into your life. Some people will marry their very first 'best friend' and stay married, but this is not common. Others will meet their 'best friend' in college and marry. Still others, the creatives and the adventurers, endure many relationships (and marriages) as a journey to figure themselves out. Some have parents who are good role models for them, but many don't. Some are confused with their sexual orientation, ultimately to decide who they are.

<u>The seven stages of LOVE from "*Marigold*":</u>

1. Attraction
2. Infatuation
3. Love
4. Reverence
5. Worship
6. Obsession
7. Death

<u>Four Rules to a Fair Fight:</u>

1. Stay on topic (don't bring in the past or other issues aka known as the kitchen sink).
2. Don't fight dirty.
3. Learn to negotiate (somethings give in).
4. Stay good humored (all things DO pass).

<u>Other Relationship Rules</u>:

1. Show sincere appreciation for each other.
2. Have date nights even after you move in together and/or get married.
3. Express how you feel by using the 'I' word vs. attacking with 'you' and putting the other person in defense.
4. Express how you feel vs. stuffing it down as your partner will sense you are upset and shutting down. They will feel your lack of trust and feel rejected as a result.
5. Find unique ways to make it work.
6. Be a good listener: eye contact, full attention, don't interrupt, and choose words carefully.
7. In areas of no apparent resolution, keep communicating and find compromise on each side.

<u>Conflict Resolution</u>:

- Create an agreed upon plan of attack for problem resolution. Set a time to deal with it (strategic planning).

Katie & Gay Hendricks have created multiple *Hearts in Harmony* programs. You can get a wealth of helpful relationship advice by subscribing to their emails.

High School

This is an exercise of contemplation. Where were you at in love and relationships when you were 13-18? And how has the experience affected you in future relationships?

Boys or Girls I Liked When I Was in High School

Friends I Had When I Was In High School

Notes to My 16-Year-Old Self

If I Were 16 Again, I'd...

When I Was 16, I Wanted To...

My Favorite Activities Were...

Salmon & Veggies

The following is for 1 serving.

Heat a small frying pan with a little coconut oil.

Add 1 filet of Frozen Alaskan Wild Caught Salmon.
(Cover and cook for 10 minutes.)

Add Frozen Broccoli and/or Cauliflower.
(Cover and cook for another 5 minutes)

Sprinkle with Himalayan pink salt or salad dressing.

Note: Recently in the news, the Sound in Washington where Salmon spawn was found to be poluted. It is better to get Salmon from Alaska waters. Avoid farm-raised salmon which is higher in Omega 6. You want more Omega 3. "Wild Caught" from China has been known to have color and flavor added, as well as be contaminated with plastic.

<u>Music I Like</u>

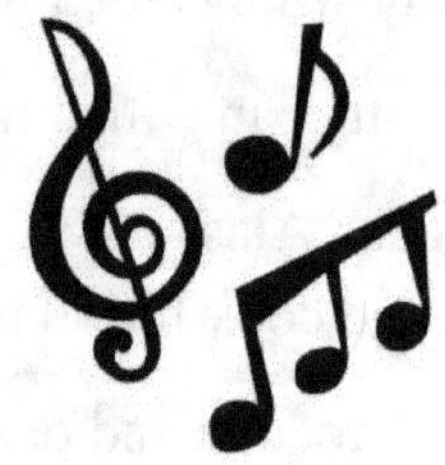

Listening to moving **music** causes the brain to release dopamine, a feel-good chemical. **People** love **music** for much the same reason they're drawn to sex, drugs, gambling, and delicious food, according to new research. (Google)

List below the music you enjoy listening to:

Tasty Quinoa

Mix ½ cup of quinoa, rinsed in a fine strainer,
with 1 cup water in a small pot.
Bring to a boil,
then lower the heat to simmer for 15 minutes.
(Simmering too high will make a boil-over mess.)
Turn heat off and let sit for an additional 10 minutes.

Add ½ TBSN ground flax seeds.
Add veggies if desired.

Add 1 TBSP salad dressing.*

Salad Dressing

Combine in a small glass mason jar:
¼ cup apple cider vinegar (organic)
¼ cup balsamic vinegar
½ cup avocado oil
1 tsp honey (optional)
(Let spoon of honey sit in mix for several hours.
The honey will dissolve.)

Age 18

Notes to My 18-Year-Old Self

When I Was 18, I Wanted To...

<u>What's Next?</u>

You graduated high school (or maybe you didn't). Did you go to college or trade school? Go to work for a family business? Start your own business? Join the military?

If you went to college, you probably took assessment tests. Understanding more about how you fit in personality wise is important. Many employers do these tests to learn more about you. Here are some tests you can take.

Human Metrics - http://www.humanmetrics.com/

Career Clusters Interest Survey (The Sixteen Career Clusters):
https://www.careerwise.mnscu.edu/careers/clusterSurvey

The Rhys Method -
http://rhysthomasinstitute.com/rhys-method-life-purpose-profiles/rhys-method-life-purpose-profiles-questionnaire/

DISC Personality Testing -
https://www.discinsights.com/

Personality Colors Quiz – https://jasonadamo.com

Note: The four categories in DISC are Dominant, Influencing, Steady, and Compliant. The Career Clusters Survey includes Feeling, Intuition, Sensing, and Thinking.

KEEP MOVING...
JUST LIKE A SQUIRREL

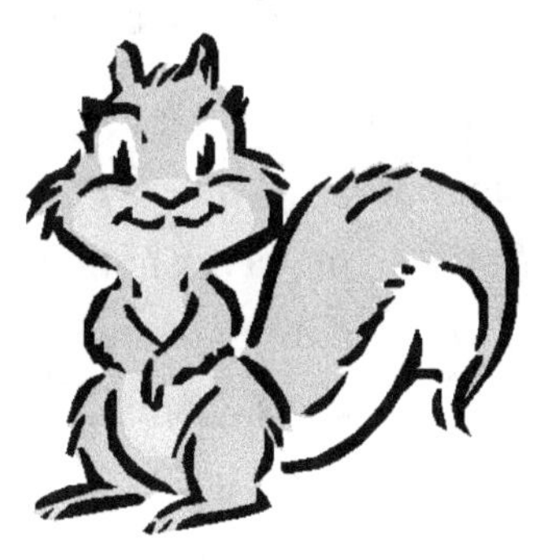

Exercise

Often times, once we graduate high school (and college), we become sedentary. Perhaps it is a desk job. Or you work 18 hours a day in sales or in your own business. Between the SAD (Standard American Diet) and lack of movement, weight gain (if it hasn't already been an issue) becomes an issue. The philosophy of exercise has evolved over the years. Now trainers are saying that doing short bursts of intense exercise often during the day is good for your heart as it trains your heart to handle stress that triggers fight or flight responses in your body. You can put work or studying on hold every two hours and do a burst of:

- Climbing up and down stairs.
- Jogging in place.
- Planks (unless you have shoulder issues).
- Push-ups (do them against a wall or counter if you have shoulder issues).
- Deep breathing.
- Some squats, lunges, etc.
- Pedal on a stationary bike. (Position a music stand in front of it for your reading material.)
- Leslie Sansone's *Walk At Home* on YouTube.
- Dancing.

Note: Most fitness centers, including the YMCA, have Personal Trainers to assist you with an exercise program catered to your body. Balance is key.

Age 21

Notes to My 21-Year Old Self

If I Were 21 Again, I'd...

Meditate

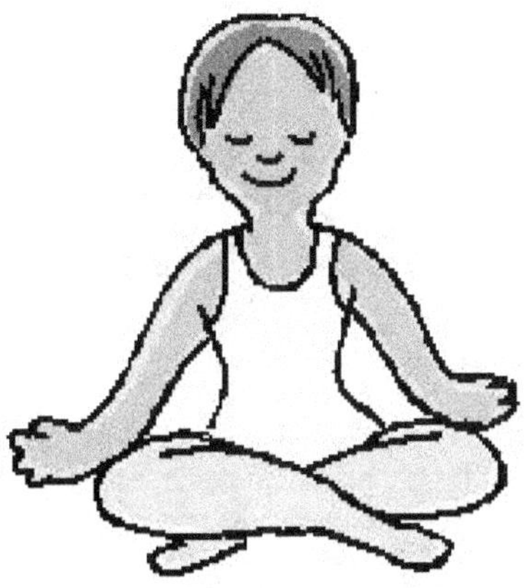

Take time out of your busy life to relax and meditate. Become aware of your posture and breathe deeply through your diaphragm. Meditation reduces anxiety and fosters positive emotions. Imagine… stagnant toxic energy draining out of the soles of your feet and into the center of the earth. Then imagine the crown of your head opening to receive the unconditional love and healing from the Creator of All That Is. Feel it fill every inch of your body. Bring this energy up from the Earth into your heart. Bring this energy from above into your heart. Visualize this energy growing stronger and stronger, expanding out from your body. Surround yourself with this love. Finally, send this love out to all your loved ones and to the entire planet. And if you believe in extraterrestrials, send some love to the entire Universe!

Friends & Social Life

People who have strong social connections are less prone to depression and other mental illnesses. Volunteering is another healthy activity as it is in the giving that you receive. List below who your current friends, social circles, and volunteer activities are.

On the other hand, if you have friends, social circles, or situations that drain your energy, it is time to…

Prune Your Bushes

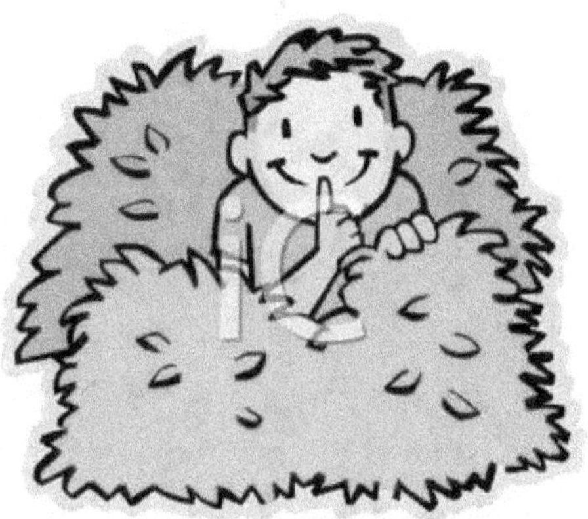

…let them go. Sometimes there are family members you should let go of, too. Draining situations and relationships will affect your health, your heart, and your mind. They will also put a damper on your ambitions. List below people and situations you need to let go of.

<table>
<tr><td>

</td></tr>
<tr><td>
</td></tr>
<tr><td>
</td></tr>
<tr><td>
</td></tr>
<tr><td>
</td></tr>
</table>

Learn Something New

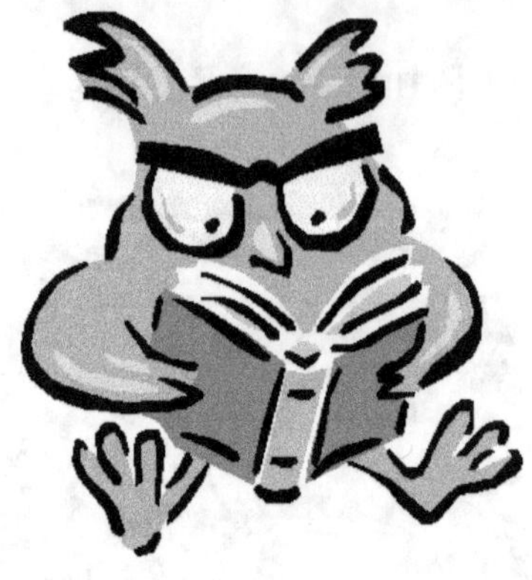

Be a lifetime student. Read books, take continuing educations classes, take advantage of free online courses. Toastmasters is a world-wide organization with local clubs that facilitate growth as well – in education, leadership, communication, speaking, and professional development.

Something New I Can Learn

<u>Passion</u>

Webster defines passion in multiple ways, including:

- Intense, driving, or overmastering feeling or conviction
- a strong liking or desire for or devotion to some activity, object, or concept
- Sexual desire
- An object of desire or deep interest

Contemplate what you are truly passionate about. What inspires you? What things do you do that fill you up with adrenaline type energy and drive similar to the feeling of being in love? Some examples include:

- Making a difference (locally or on the planet)
- Starting my own business
- Writing
- Playing musical instrument / Singing
- Prayer worship
- Working with children
- Teaching / mentoring

Write what inspires passion for you.

BE YOUR OWN BEST FRIEND!

You always have to
remember to take care
of yourself first and
foremost, because
when you stop taking
care of yourself you get
out of balance and you
really forget how to
take care of others.

Jada Pinkett Smith

Self-Care

Ladies: I mentioned avoiding toxic toothpaste in *Rise and Shine!* Also use caution in what products you use if you are gluten sensitive, but I must also mention dousing yourselves with products that have formaldehyde and other toxins are hazardous to your health. You probably have watched a LOT of commercials that promote great products… but just like you don't get the whole story when they advertise pharmaceutical drugs, you are not getting the whole story of what is in these products. I don't know about you, but I used to buy inexpensive self-care products for YEARS before I found out what is in them.

Men: Did you know? The cologne you use every morning when you shave could be lowering your testosterone.

If you haven't done so already, you may want to consider getting a filter for your shower. Besides chlorine, there are other toxins coming in through your water. Some people install expensive filter systems in their homes that covers everything, but you can also get gadget specific filters for faucets and shower heads.

The Environmental Working Group (ewg.org) has an extensive website with information about: what's in your tap water, shampoo, antibacterial products, cleaners, the pesticides in your food, GMOs, and more.

In addition to reading up on political news (if this is your thing), read up on food, health, and finance news.

Places I Want to Go / Travel

TREASURE YOUR TIME

TREASURE YOUR CONNECTIONS

TREASURE YOUR MEMORIES

EVERY CATERPILLAR GOES
THROUGH GROWING PAINS
BEFORE IT EMERGES FROM A
COCOON AS A BEAUTIFUL
BUTTERFLY.

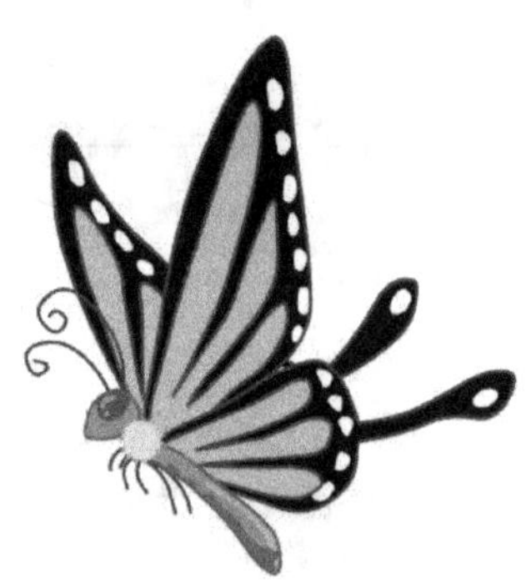

If I Could Do Anything, I'd...

Turkey Stew

In a large crock pot:

Two turkey thighs or other turkey pieces (even turkey necks are great for stew)

Water

Cilantro

Parsley

Optional: Trader Joe's 21 Seasoning Salute or other favorite spices.

Cook on high for one – two hours.

Add:

Harmony House or fresh:

Onion, Carrots, Cabbage, Baby Bok Choy

Cook on low for one – two more hours.

Keep warm and graze all afternoon and evening.

Refrigerate leftovers.

Note: Add a whole acorn squash or sweet potatoes to eat later. Also, use chicken instead of turkey if desired. Choose turkey and chicken raised without hormones and antibiotics, preferably pasture raised.

The Art of Manifesting

You were incarnated with IMAGINATION. Do you know how to use it? I'm sure you used your imagination all the time when you were a child. The ability is still there.

Without conscious awareness, you are continuously uploading thoughts into your brain. Then your brain (and the Universe) conspires to manifest your life based on these thoughts.

An earlier exercise was based on keeping track of your thoughts and becoming aware of any cognitive distortions you may have. The next two exercises are for imagining you have unlimited resources and potential.

If I had the money, I'd…

Charities / Non-Profits I'd donate to…

Make the list LONG. Include in your imagined abundance substantial giving, even if it is service and volunteering vs. donating money.

Volunteering and service is also good for your mental health. See Strong Social Connections.

If I Had the Money, I'd...

Charities / Non-Profits I'd Donate To...

Meals On The Run

Whatever you do, avoid the fast food chains. There is NOTHING in the food you really should be eating. Refer to the Basic Nutrition page. Especially, avoid fried food!

Google facts about the rising obesity and diabesity in our country. It's hard to believe so many people are completely unaware of how the food they eat affects their health.

Cook one pot meals in a crockpot and take leftovers. Get yourself one or more insulated bags to carry food in. If you must, it is better to stop at a grocery store and get fresh produce. Watch the premade salads if they come with dressing with one of the oils to avoid.

Here are some alternative ideas for a meal on the run.

Dried Fruit + Raw Nuts

Hard-boiled egg(s) + carrot sticks

Base Culture Nutty Pumpkin Bread Mini Bar

Leftovers or premade salad

Egg Loaf (see recipe)

Homemade Organic Smoothie

Hydrate Harmony House veggies like cabbage, carrot, and onion in a small canning jar. Add almond slivers and homemade salad dressing.

Stop at a health food store or restaurant.

Beef Stew

In a large crockpot – high setting – 1 hour:

Grass Fed Organic (ground) Beef

Water

Spices

One or more whole beets

After an hour, turn to low setting and add:

Onion, Carrots, & Celery (fresh or Harmony House)

Fresh Mushrooms

About 1/3 of a head of cabbage

Simmer on low for about 2 more hours

Note: Add a whole Acorn Squash in the beginning and you won't have to cut through this very hard squash. Let cool and enjoy for another meal!

Complimentary & Alternative Medicine

Medicine is like politics and religion. There are many modalities, beliefs, and viewpoints.

Educate yourself so you can make intelligent decisions.

By the time symptoms show up in your body, they have already been there energetically, which can be seen with Kirlian cameras. Wouldn't it make more sense to look for the energetic imbalances that started the entire cascade of events? And begin at the beginning with nutrition and stress management?

Most doctors only received an hour of education on nutrition in medical school. What they ARE taught is to prescribe the drugs the pharmaceutical industries have told them to prescribe. These companies are known to falsify reports just to get their drugs into the market – it's all about the profits to them. They even pay commission to doctors who prescribe them.

Before you choose to go the pharmaceutical route for drugs that are for your SYMPTOMS, become your own health detective/advocate and search for the root cause. All the drugs with side effects will keep you going back for more tests and more drugs. Most of the tests and imaging are merely tools for drug prescribing and extensive medical treatments.

Here is a list of some of the alternative practitioners who can help you find this root cause – and correct them with nutrition and other alternative modalities. Sadly, most insurance doesn't cover these services, but all the mainstream docs are trained to keep you sick so they can stay in business. If you work for an organization that has health savings accounts, you may find in the long run, your medical care to cost less.

- Functional Medicine / Naturopathic Medicine
- Nutrition / Kinesiology / Muscle Testing
- Acupuncture / Chinese Medicine
- Myotherapy / Massage / Cranial Sacral Therapy
- Chiropractic
- Energy Medicine / Reiki / Bioenergetics
- Homeopathy / Bach Flower Remedies
- Essential Oils
- Cognitive Behavioral Therapy
- Energy and Positive Psychology
- Life Coaches
- Health Coaches / Personal Trainers
- EFT / NLP / Theta Healing

Tests you can get on your own:

Mineral Hair Analysis –
https://www.aurorahealthandnutrition.com/

The Shomon Autoimmune Disease Profile & Complete
Thyroid Panel –
https://thyroid-info.mymedlab.com/mary-shomon-
profiles/shomon-autoimmune-profile

For info about BioTerrain testing: -
http://www.mybodyofknowledge.net/bioterrain-
assessment.html

For info about Bioenergetics: -
https://en.wikipedia.org/wiki/Bioenergetics

Website to find a Naturopathic Physician –
http://www.naturopathic.org/

Reading List for Health

CFS Unravelled by Dan Neuffer

Feeling Good: The New Mood Therapy by David D. Burns, M.D.

Heal Your Pain Now by Joe Tatta, DPT, CNS

One Spirit Medicine by Alberto Villoldo, Ph.D.

Reinventing The Body, Resurrecting The Soul by Deepak Chopra

Solving the Autoimmune Puzzle: The Woman's Guide to Reclaiming Emotional Freedom and Vibrant Health by Dr. Keesha Ewers

The Autoimmune Fix by Tom O'Bryan, DC, CCN, DACBN

The Biology of Belief by Bruce Lipton, Ph.D.

The Body Keeps The Score by Bessel Van Der Kolk, M.D.

Transforming Anxiety by Doc Childre & Deborah Rozman, Ph.D.

What Should I Do With My Life? by Po Bronson

Younger Next Year by Chris Crowley & Henry S. Lodge, M.D.

Health Goals- Practitioners

Faith

Faith is powerful. Prayer is powerful. What is even more powerful is TRUST that there is a power greater than everything, and when you BELIEVE you DESERVE what you ask for, you will receive it. LOVE every part of yourself as God loves you and FORGIVE yourself for all the things you said or didn't say as well as the decisions you made that resulted in poor outcomes. Release all anger and resentment you have toward what happened to you. It isn't easy, but it can be done.

Faith comes in all shapes, sizes, and nationalities. There are as many beliefs as there are people even though there are basic categories of religion. It doesn't really matter WHAT you believe in (except if it is centered around hell and damnation which was man-made to control the masses), it only matters that you believe in a power greater than everything. Some people call this power The Creator of All That Is.

The only true religion is LOVE. Make love the center of your life. Remember: your cells are affected by your thoughts, beliefs, and environment. Learn about all the religions of the world, open your mind, and you'll see the base of all of them is LOVE. When you learn more about other people and nationalities, your world will expand.

Books to read:

The History of God by Karen Armstrong

Finding God by John H. Clark III

Mid-Life

Many people face major changes when they are about 40 years old. These changes can include a new marriage, divorce, death, empty nest, a housewife who decides to go to work, major career changes, go back to college for a degree, or even disability. Where are you at with life / work / career? Explore every possibility! There is a huge world out there!

AARP has a program called *Life Reimagined* which can help you figure out what to do next in life. Or perhaps you have already figured out what you want to do next.

There are many online classes in a variety of subjects plus unlimited YouTube videos on just about every topic. Here are some websites you can check out.

MIT Open Courseware - http://ocw.mit.edu/index.htm

Quizlet - https://quizlet.com/

Savelle Assessment:
https://www.savilleassessment.com/career-guidance-and-self-development

Uma Girish (Grief Guide) - https://umagirish.com/

THERE IS MORE LIFE TO LIVE -

DREAM BIG AND GO FOR IT!

When I am 50 Years Old...

...or what I want to tell my 50-year-old self

When I am 60 Years Old...

...or what I want to tell my 60-year-old self

<u>Aging</u>

Strong Social Connections

Strong social connections continue to be vital as you age. There are many clubs and organizations you can get involved in at some level. It doesn't have to be church, although many are active in their religious organizations.

Clubs / Organizations to consider:

- In Texas, there is the Texas Education Extension Association
- Toastmasters (there is no age limit)
- Local health club and/or pool
- Volunteering at the Chamber of Commerce
- Meetup groups (Meetup.com)
- Senior Center
- Local Animal Shelters
- Libraries and Art Guilds
- Community Colleges (clubs and continued ed)

Organizations/Clubs I can get involved in:

When I am 70 Years Old...

When I am 80 Years Old...

When I am 90 Years Old...

Final Arrangements

The only one who knows how long we have on earth is our Creator. It is so important to have final arrangements prepared in advance which entails much more than a life insurance policy. And the costs for burial and funeral arrangements continue to rise.

If cremation is your thing, find a local funeral home or crematorium that can sell you a prepaid cremation package, insured through the state you live in. This package should include everything you want your family and/or loved ones to know, including the eulogy you want spoken and where you want your ashes to be released. Be sure to shop around. Consider getting a supplement that will cover expenses should you leave the planet while traveling (travelassuranceplan.com).

For info about pre-paid plans, here's an article you can read: http://www.elderlawanswers.com/pre-paid-funeral-plans-buyer-beware-1098

A will can only contain information on the transfer of 'tangible' property such as a house, car, jewelry, bank accounts, stock, etc. To avoid sibling rivalry on all accounts, it is best to know ahead of time what everyone would want when you depart. You can make a scrapbook of photos and circulate it so everyone can reserve items they want. If more than one person wants the same item, it is best to work this out while you are still HERE. This is especially essential where family heirlooms are concerned.

How do you want to be remembered? Like authors have a bio, you can write up your accomplishments and anything else you want to be remembered for.

Do you want a gathering with a memorial picture board? A celebration of life? If you are not going to be cremated, do you want open or closed casket?

Do you want a ceremony with religious or spiritual overtones? A traditional funeral? Who do you want to say your eulogy? Your church pastor or minister? A loved one? Do you want to write your own eulogy in advance? What music do you want played?

There is a movie about two young people who know they are dying. They decide to have a relationship anyway knowing how painful it will be when one of them goes first. They plan their whole funeral and have it while they are still living. It was a tear-jerker, but wonderful!

You should also have an Advanced Healthcare Directive/Medical Power of Attorney on file with your doctor and designated family member. In addition to a Medical Power of Attorney, you may also need a Durable Financial Power of Attorney to designate someone who is authorized to handle your financial affairs should you become incapacitated mentally or physically.

Note: Prepaid cremation packages from Neptune Society are high-priced. You can get less expensive ones locally or through the military (if you served). I found a family-owned operation which charges less than the local funeral home.

Tips on Organizing

Organizing Your Life: There are many ways to do this. You can use a Google Doc and organize everything in a single document you can view from your phone. Or create a folder in your Google Drive for separate Google Docs for each topic. A second option is using one of many task apps on your phone. A third option is a loose-leaf binder with pocket dividers similar to what I suggest for keeping your finances organized. A fourth option is using a journal.

Email: Keep your email inbox empty by creating priority folders with the @ sign in front of topics like @Action, @Bills to Pay, and @Orders Pending. These folders will appear at the top of your list of folders. File the rest of the emails you want to save in additional email folders. Delete the rest of your emails. This helps with the feeling of overwhelm when you open your emails.

Finance: I suggest a three-ring binder and clear (colored) divider pages with pockets. After using the Monthly Cash Flow Plan in an upcoming section to pencil in your current numbers, use a digital spread-sheet (MS Excel or Google Sheets) to plug in all your numbers and adjust them as needed, using a formula calculate your totals. Print off a new one each month. In section 1, include this budget and your check register. Your bills for the current month will go in the front pocket. If your financial life is more complex, here are additional pockets and sections to include:

➢ Pending orders & copies of recurring expenses.
➢ Medical (If you are making payments, use ledger sheets to track them. Insert current bills into pocket.)
➢ A section that includes current Social Security statements and other related documents.
➢ Future Planning & miscellaneous records.

Ground Mail: When you collect your mail, pull out the bills and put them in the bills-to-pay folder of your finance binder. If you get paid once a month, put it all in the same folder with a printout of the budget you will make (included later in this book). If you get paid weekly (or biweekly) write on multiple folders which bills go in them – a folder for due the 1st, one for due the 15th, etc.

Wardrobe: Marie Condo is quite famous for her book: *The Life-Changing Magic of Tidying Up*. She helps people get a grip on having too many clothes, shoes, and other stuff. In the meantime, you can experiment with holding pieces up to your heart. If your body falls forward, keep it. If it falls back, don't. You can take photos of your outfits with your smartphone. This will come in handy when you are shopping for something to add to what you already have and when you have foggy brain in the morning and forget which pieces go together. You can also keep a list of outfits.

Kitchen & Other Rooms: There are umpteen different sizes of baskets you can use in your refrigerator, freezer, and cabinets to keep food organized by what it is. You can take the entire basket out to find what you need vs. food getting shoved to the back and forgotten. In my refrigerator, I have two baskets for prepared food, a basket for apples and other fruit, and a basket for nuts and miscellaneous. In the freezer, I have four baskets: one for unopened packages of frozen vegetables, one for open packages of frozen vegetables, one for fish and other meat, and one for ice packs. Use baskets on bookshelves, too, to organize toys, office supplies, purses, shoes, etc.

Time Management: There are numerous time management tools available, and I've tried many. To avoid using a huge calendar, I decided I didn't need to save all that data aka to-do lists. I found a simple TASKS app I have on my phone that handles both appointments and important tasks very conveniently. This app includes dates and descriptions in addition to the title of the task, so I include appointments with the time in front of it. I love this app because if it is something I do on a regular basis, once I've done it, I open it and move it to the next date. If I don't have time to complete a task, I can move it to another date.

Articles: Pinterest is awesome when it comes to collecting and organizing digital articles you find on the internet. But what do you do with all the articles you are saving from Magazines? Or ones you've printed out? Get colored D-ring binders and organize your articles according to subject! For instance, a Pink binder for articles about Relationships and Parenting. Green for articles and paperwork pertaining to Life Purpose-Goals-Income Earning Opportunities. White for Current Medical Records, organized with tabs for Blood Tests, Receipts, Vision, Dental, Tests (Bone Scan, X-Rays, Colonoscopy, etc.)

Sleep

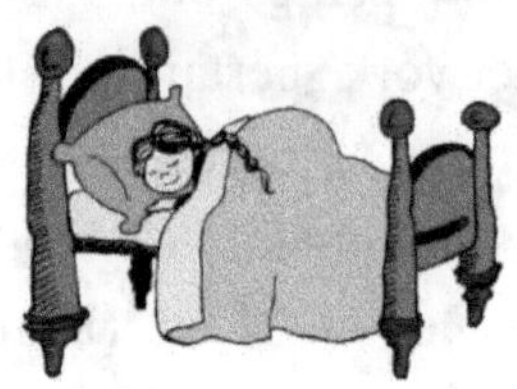

What are your sleep patterns? Do you feel like you are getting enough sleep? Some people can get by on five hours, but other people need as much as nine.

Sleep is essential as this is the time the body regenerates and heals. People with Fibromyalgia and other chronic (pain) conditions don't get the REM sleep they need so they wake up tired and achy.

People who snore may have sleep apnea (like I do), so they don't get enough oxygen when they sleep. Lack of oxygen spills over into achy muscles and other health conditions.

Years of drinking Pepsi, coffee, and caffeinated drinks takes a toll on your heart and adrenals. You stay on continuous fight or flight mode. Humans were not created to function this way. Eventually, you will crash – and the crash may be while you're driving.

Sleeping potions and pharmaceuticals have side effects, often leaving you with a hangover – so you then need something else to jump start you the next morning.

Helpful: Diffuse Lavender Essential Oil in an Ultrasonic Diffuser. Listen to "white noise."

Take Time Out To Play

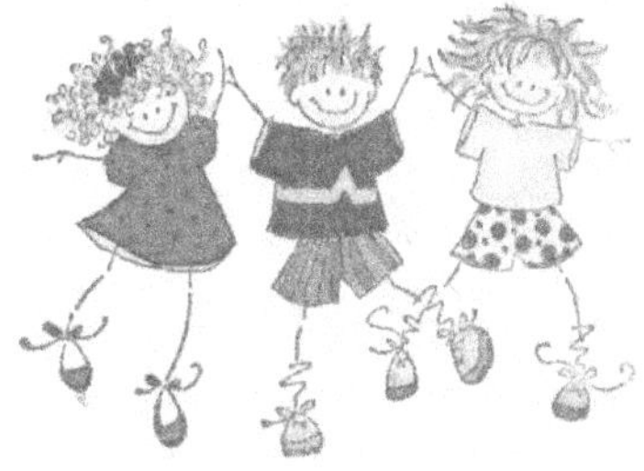

Newspapers, Television, Radio, and Social Media are filled with all the awful things that are happening in our world. The media have limited time and space for news, and what they report are influenced by those with money and power. Commercials are paid for by the organizations with money – and most of what they televise is not good for us, including the pharmaceuticals and foods that have toxic ingredients. Even our children are targeted for ads.

Remember to take time out to PLAY, and choose to focus on all the good – there really is quite a bit of it. Our positive intentions CAN make a difference! Focus on what you can be grateful for. Attitude makes or breaks a person's psyche.

> ## BELIEVE THERE IS GOOD
> ## IN THIS WORLD

YOUR PHYSICAL BODY IS
NOT A MATERIAL THING,
IT'S AN ACTIVITY IN YOUR
OWN CONSCIOUSNESS.

Deepak Chopra

Finance

Things we should have learned in high school:

- How to create a budget & balance a checkbook
- The importance of having an emergency fund
- The cost of credit & loans
- The cost of instant gratification
- How to buy or lease a car
- Contracts (and the fine print)
- How your credit can affect employment
- Parenting (financial planning)

This next section includes a cash flow worksheet. It may be helpful to plug the numbers into an Excel or Google Sheet and have the totals automatically calculate. This way, you can easily adjust your numbers to make sure your expenses don't exceed your income.

It's a good idea to withdraw the cash for groceries and other incidentals vs. using a debit card to avoid accidently or unknowingly overspending.

If you have credit card debt, it is a good idea to split the funds left after household and fixed expenses 50/50 to pay down debt and establish an emergency fund.

Abundance isn't just about money. It is a mindset. Be sure to practice gratitude and become aware of the abundance of what you DO have vs. dwelling on what you don't.

<u>Books to read on finance</u>:
Unshakeable by Tony Robbins
The Finish Rich Workbook by Richard Bach
The Soul of Money by Lynne Twist
Books by Dave Ramsey (Financial Peace University)

Monthly Cash Flow Plan

Net Take-Home Pay / Other Income ____________

Monthly Expenses ____________

Difference ____________

Monthly Expense Detail

(10%)   Savings and Investments
              Pension plans
              IRA's   ____________
              Emergency fund   ____________

(22%)   Housing Costs
              Mortgage Payment/Rent   ____________
              Property Taxes   ____________
              Property or Renter's Insurance   ____________
              Home Equity Loan   ____________

(18%)   Consumer Debt
              Department Store Accounts   ____________
              Credit Cards   ____________
              Bank Loans   ____________
              Car Payment(s)   ____________
              Other Time Payments   ____________

(50%)   Other Monthly Expenses*
              Child Support/Alimony   ____________
              Electricity   ____________
              Gas   ____________
              Water   ____________

Auto Insurance _______________

Life Insurance _______________

Medical _______________

Dental _______________

Vision _______________

Other Insurance _______________

Groceries _______________

Gasoline/Diesel _______________

Car Maintenance _______________

Entertainment _______________

TV / Internet / Cell Phone _______________

Clothing _______________

Vacation _______________

School Tuition _______________

School Supplies _______________

Organization Dues _______________

Subscriptions _______________

Household Items _______________

Miscellaneous _______________

Total Expenses _______________

*This area may have to be slashed to allow for savings and investments and overruns in other areas. If monies used for "other monthly expenses" represent less than 50% of total take-home pay, other areas can be expanded—i.e. purchasing a bigger home or increasing the savings and investing portion.

Notes:

____

____

____

Birthdays & Anniversaries

JANUARY

FEBRUARY

MARCH

APRIL

MAY

JUNE

JULY

AUGUST

SEPTEMBER

OCTOBER

NOVEMBER

DECEMBER

<u>Menu Planning</u>

Breakfasts:

Lunches

Dinners

Master Shopping List

Protein (Meat, Fish, etc.)	Dairy / Non-Dairy
Fruit	Vegetables
Nuts / Seeds	Condiments
Supplements	Paper Products

Abundance!

<u>Abundance Journal</u>

Believe it or not, when you keep track of every little thing that shows up in your life, including pennies on the ground, your focus switches to abundance. The more you write down in this category, the more shows up. It gets pretty exciting!

Gratitude Journal

Here you will grow your list of what you are grateful for. The more you focus on Gratitude, the less you will focus on the opposite. Your mind can't be in both places at the same time. Even grief support coaches suggest this exercise to get past the initial paralysis of grief. Keep in mind, that ANYTHING that dies can catapult you into grief. The end of a relationship or marriage, losing a job, developing a disability, and housing changes affect a person just as powerfully as when someone dies.

Here are three people who have moved past grief to transform their lives and help others.

Linda Bocanegra: After the loss of her son, Linda wrote *Waking Up To The Loving World of Spirt* and does seminars on grief recovery. You can find her book on Amazon.
http://www.wakinguptothelovingworldofspirit.com/

Uma Girish: After the loss of her mother, Uma wrote *Losing Amma, Finding Home* which started her on a path as a Grief Guide, Author, and Dream Coach. She travels the world giving seminars. You can find her book on Amazon. https://umagirish.com/

Kelly Buckley: After the loss of her son, Kelly created JOLT, *Just One Little Thing*, launching an online community which has a loyal following worldwide. You can find her book on Amazon.
http://www.kellybuckley.com

Write every little thing you can be grateful for. If you need some help, Kelly has a Facebook community where you can get support. Include synchronicities you notice.

115

Self Portrait

Who am I today?
What characteristics do I admire about myself?

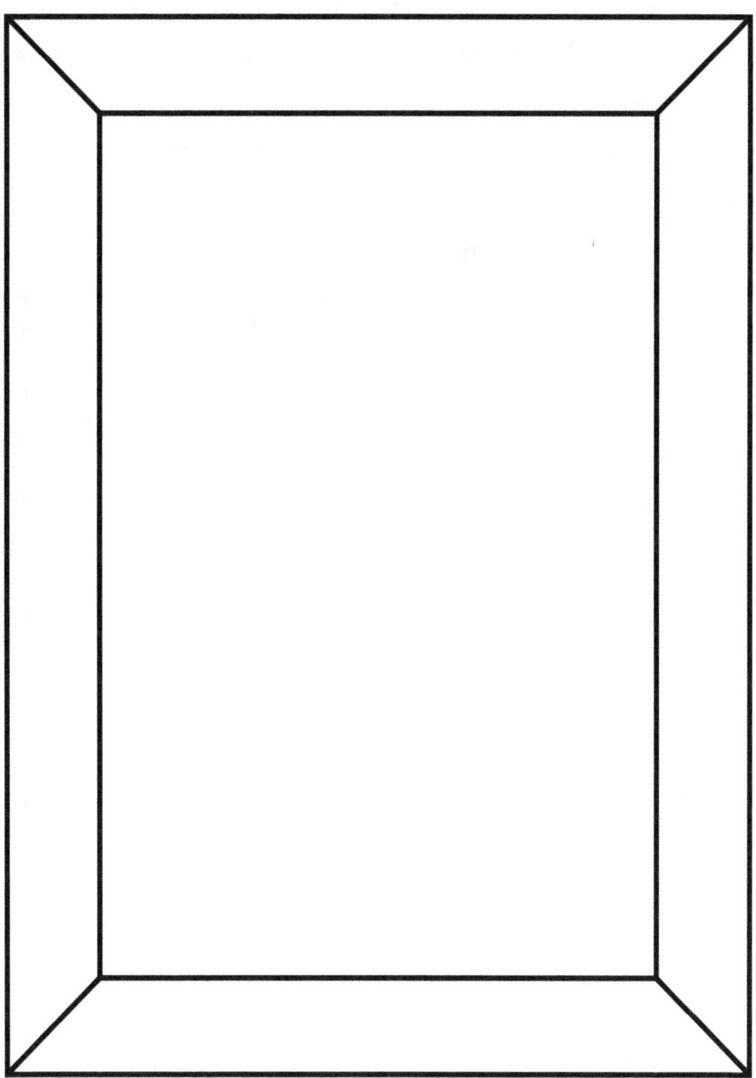

Brain Dumping Page #1

Brain dumping is a term used to describe writing down anything that comes up in your mind about a particular subject. For example, "My New Book" would include chapter titles, characters phrases, ideas, you would like to include.

<u>Brain Dumping Page #2</u>

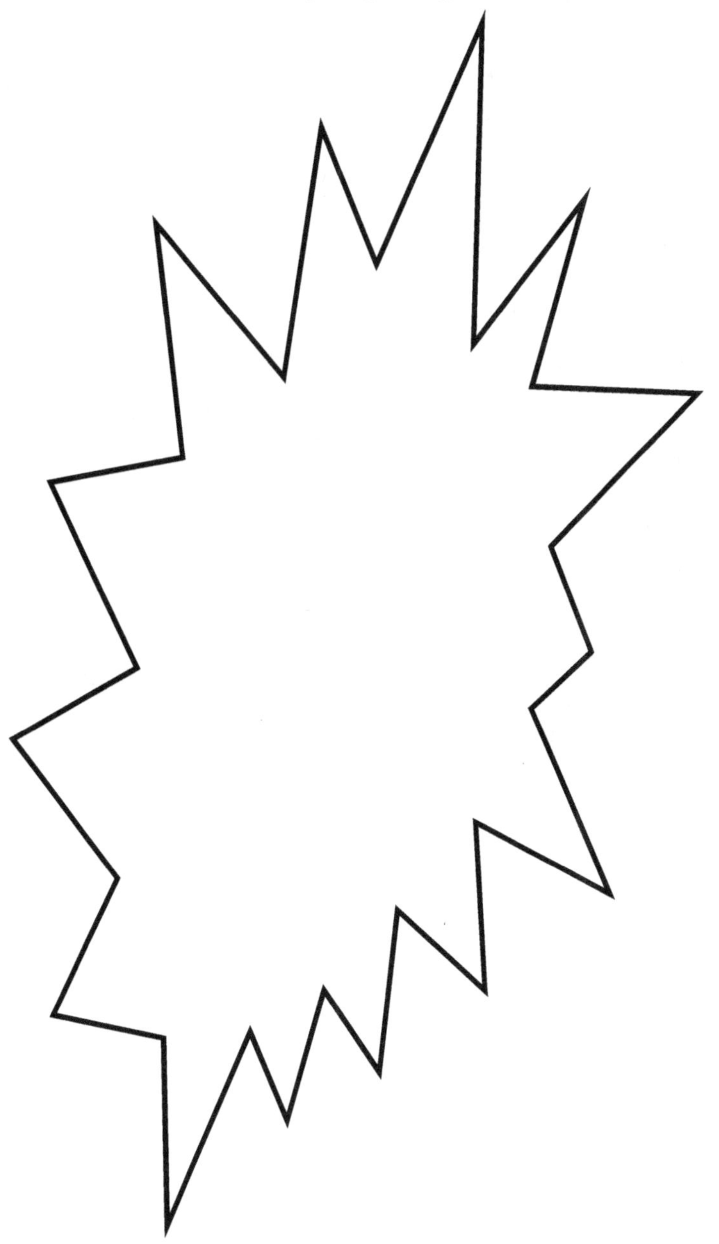

Brain Dumping Page #3

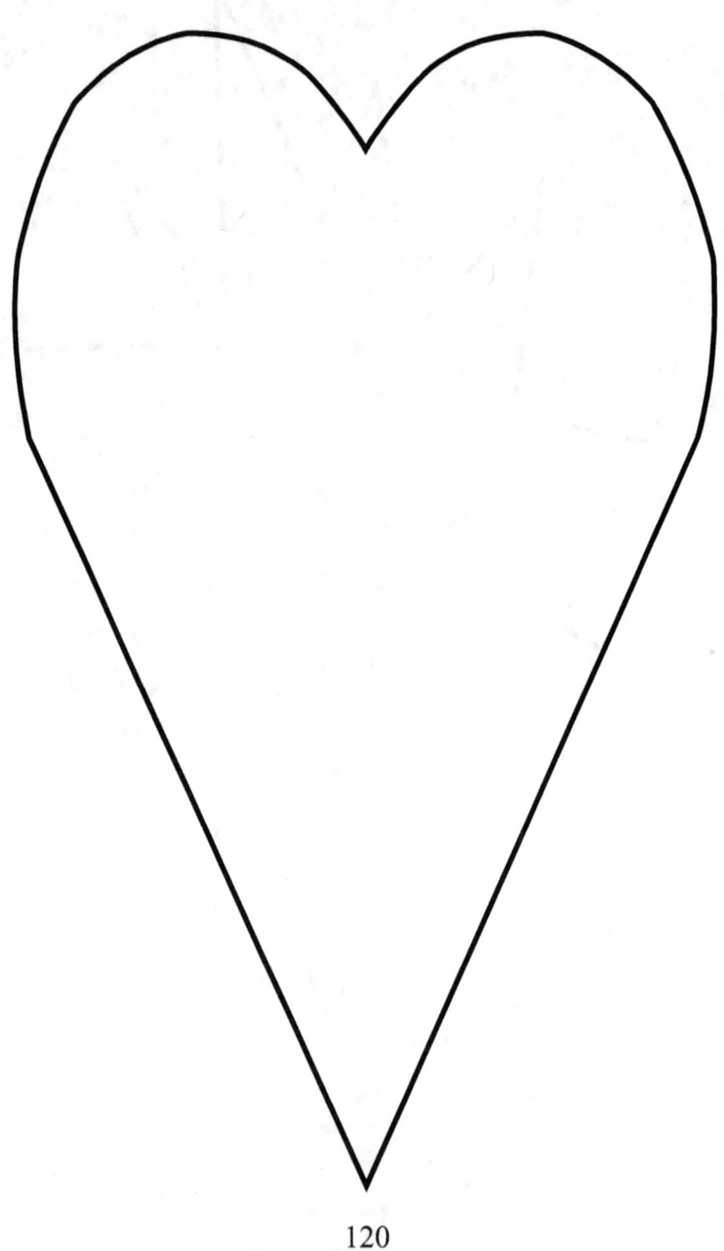

Notes

Index

I hoped you found this journal just the tool you needed to move forward in living an amazing life. Please take a moment to leave a review on Amazon.

amazon.com/author/reneealter

You can contact me through my website. Use the contact form in the right column. If you are using a cellphone, scroll to the bottom and click on View web version to see the form.

www.reneealtersatmosphere.com

Other Books by Renee Alter

Appearances: A Journey of Self-Discovery

Reflections: A Toolbox of Poetry

Love, Life, & God: Getting Past the Pain

View From A Tree

Creating A Meaningful Life After Disability: Posts From My Blog

Blog Therapy: Posts From My Blog Part 2

Miracles Sandwiched Between the Challenges: Making It Through The Roller Coasters Of My Life With The Help Of My Guardian Angels (Short Story)

Growing An Internal Garden to Cope With Chronic Pain, Illness, & Depression

Alternative Realities: Daydreams of Conversations

The Land of Mark (Short Story-Kindle & Audible)

The Adventures of Gnat (Short Story-Kindle & Audible)

Twin Flame (Short Story-Kindle & Audible)

Blogging A Path To The Future: Posts From My Blog Part 3

Living With Symptomatic Spondylolisthesis

Lessons From Nature

On the Move: Autobiography of a Survivor

Metamorphosis: Posts From My Blog Part 4